CROWNING GLORY

EMBRACING YOUR
NATURAL HAIR JOURNEY

LAQUITA COPELAND

Published by

Copeland Publications Group
6455 Argyle Forest Blvd Ste 21
Jacksonville, FL 32244
http://myhairlyfe.com

This book is a work of empowerment dedicated to celebrating natural beauty and uplifting everyone everywhere. The information provided within is intended to inspire and educate, supporting each reader on their unique natural hair journey.

Cover art: © LaQuita Copeland
Created and printed in the United States of America.
10 9 8 7 6 5 4 3 2 1

CONTENTS

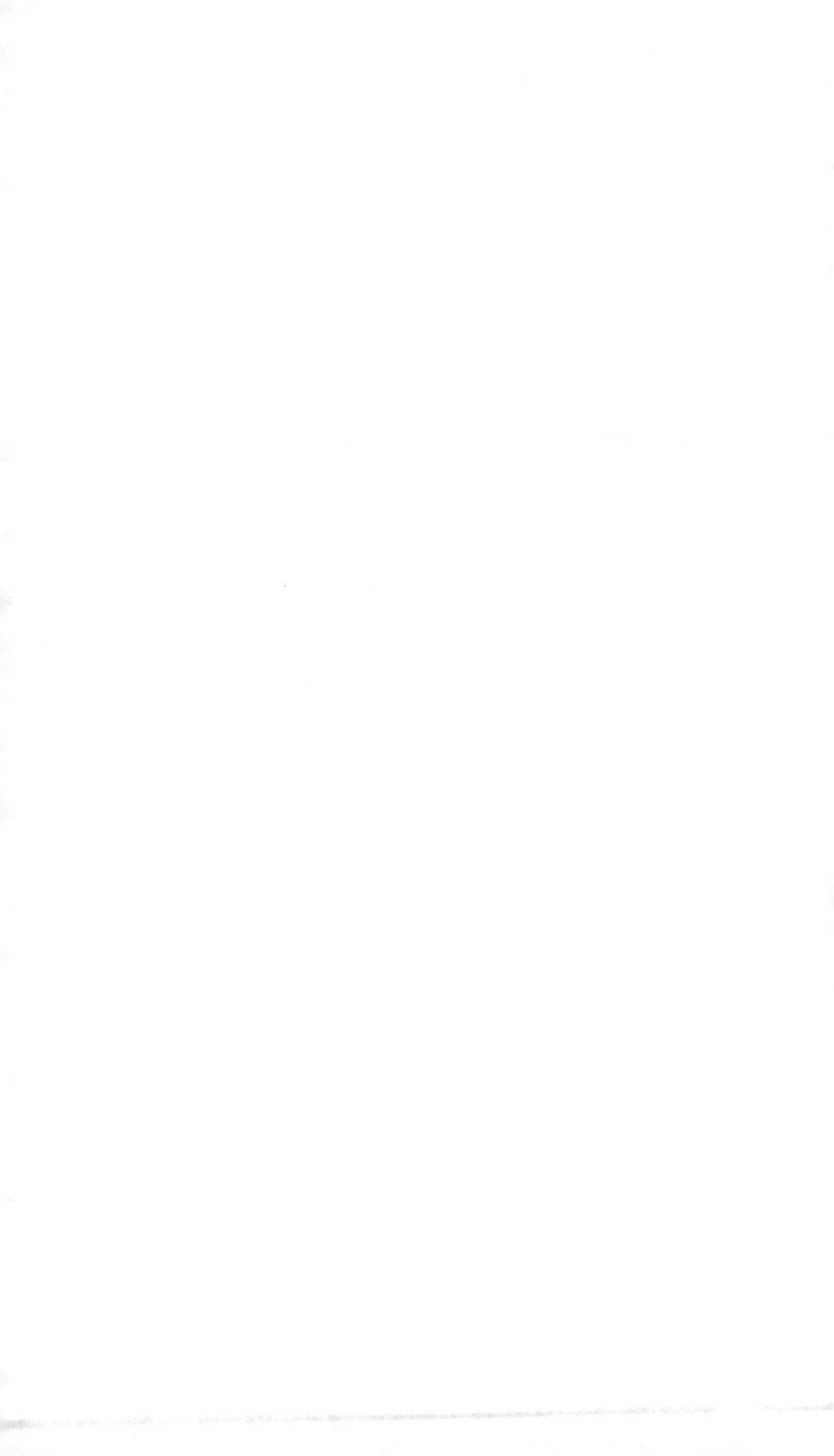

ACKNOWLEDGMENTS

A heartfelt thank you to my family, friends, and supporters. Your unwavering support and loyalty have been the driving force behind my strength and perseverance. Your presence in my life has inspired me to reach new heights, and I am profoundly grateful for the light and love you've brought to this journey. I hold each of you in high regard and deeply appreciate your role in this incredible path.

To those whose kindness and steadfastness have uplifted me along the way, my gratitude knows no bounds. Your encouragement has been a pillar of strength, guiding me through each step of this journey. Your contributions are treasured, and your presence is a gift that I cherish every day.

To everyone who has walked this path with me, your unwavering faith in my vision has ignited my passion and emboldened me to pursue my dreams. Your belief has pushed me toward excellence, and for that, I am endlessly thankful. The impact of your support has shaped this journey in profound ways.

Finally, I extend my deepest thanks to all who have encouraged and stood by me. Your dedication has been my constant motivation, inspiring me to reach beyond limits and never settle. I see you; I honor you, and I am forever grateful for the part you've played in this remarkable experience.

Your support has not only fueled my journey but has also created a ripple effect of empowerment and inspiration that extends beyond me. Each word of encouragement and every act of kindness have not gone unnoticed; they have all contributed to a tapestry of resilience that defines this endeavor. Together, we are part of a larger community that celebrates individuality, creativity, and the beauty of embracing one's authentic self.

As I continue to navigate this path, I am reminded that this journey is not just mine alone—it belongs to everyone who dares to embrace their uniqueness and share their stories. Let us uplift each other as we forge ahead, creating spaces that empower and inspire. Together, we can cultivate a legacy of self-love and pride that resonates deeply within our communities and beyond.

In closing, I invite you to join me in celebrating our collective journeys. May we continue to shine brightly, encouraging one another to dream big, embrace our natural beauty, and live authentically. Your presence in my life is a treasure, and I look forward to sharing this empowering journey with you all as we embrace our true selves. Thank you for being a part of this incredible adventure.

PROLOGUE

Welcome to *Crowning Glory: Embracing Your Natural Hair Journey*, a luxurious celebration of authenticity, empowerment, and the radiant beauty that lies in embracing your true self. This book is far more than a simple guide to hair care—it's a tribute to the strength, resilience, and cultural legacy embedded in every strand of natural hair. In a world where beauty standards have often been imposed on us, *Crowning Glory* empowers you to reclaim your narrative, embracing the fullness of your natural beauty with pride and confidence.

At HairLyfe, we view natural hair as a crown—a symbol of self-expression, individuality, and cultural heritage. Each curl, coil, and kink are a testament to empowerment, strength, and the stories we carry. This book is crafted to accompany you on your unique natural hair journey, offering expert advice, luxurious product insights, and inspiration to nurture both your hair and your self-confidence.

As you explore these pages, you'll find a wealth of knowledge on caring for your crown with love and intention. Each chapter highlights how to enhance your hair's health and beauty through the finest natural ingredients. *Crowning Glory* reflects HairLyfe's unwavering commitment to uplifting women everywhere, honoring the magnificence of natural hair in its purest, most authentic form.

This journey is not just about hair—it's about self-love and embracing your heritage. It's deeply personal to me, as it was inspired by my family's experiences, particularly my aunt's inspiring journey of hair regrowth after her battle with cancer. Her strength became the heart of HairLyfe, and this book embodies that same spirit of resilience and rebirth.

I have poured my heart into every word, every product, and every chapter of this book with the hope that it becomes a source of inspiration for you. My desire is for *Crowning Glory* to empower you to embrace your natural beauty without apology, to honor your hair as the crown that it is, and to remind you of the power that lies within.

Your natural hair is your crown, your glory, and your story—wear it with pride and grace, for it is uniquely yours.

LaQuita Copeland
Founder, HairLyfe

WELCOME TO YOUR NATURAL HAIR JOURNEY

Embrace the powerful movement of the natural hair journey—a celebration that is both timeless and profound. For Black women, natural hair transcends mere aesthetics; it serves as a cultural emblem, a bridge to our ancestral roots, and a vibrant expression of self-love and pride. Each strand embodies our rich history, narrating tales of strength, resilience, and the beauty inherent in our heritage.

At HairLyfe, we honor and celebrate your unique beauty, championing the message that embracing your natural hair is an act of empowerment. Our exquisite range of natural hair care products is thoughtfully designed to nourish and rejuvenate your hair from within, reflecting our belief that your hair is not just an adornment but a crown to be revered daily. This book serves as a comprehensive guide to unlocking the true potential of your natural hair, and we are delighted to accompany you on this empowering journey.

As you embark on this transformative path, recognize that your natural hair story is both intimate and shared by countless women rediscovering their inherent strength and beauty. *Crowning Glory* stands ready to inspire and equip you, offering valuable insights and practical tools that allow your hair to flourish as a testament to your resilience and self-love.

Let this journey be a source of empowerment as you explore the depths of your identity through your hair. The act of embracing your natural texture is a bold declaration of self-acceptance, inviting you to celebrate your individuality and the unique qualities that define you. With each chapter, you will uncover the knowledge and resources necessary to nurture not only your hair but also your confidence and self-worth.

In this sacred space, we encourage you to cultivate a mindset of love and appreciation for your hair. Understand that your natural beauty is a gift to be celebrated, and through this journey, you will forge a deeper connection with yourself and your heritage. As you delve into the pages ahead, may you find inspiration, joy, and empowerment in the journey of embracing your authentic self.

Together, let us illuminate the beauty of our natural hair, recognizing it as a symbol of strength, pride, and heritage. This journey is yours—embrace it fully, celebrate it boldly, and let your hair shine as the glorious crown it is. Welcome to a world where your true self reigns supreme, and may this journey inspire you to wear your crown with confidence and grace.

CHAPTER ONE

THE POWER OF NATURAL HAIR

Key Topics

- The historical and cultural significance of natural hair for Black women.

- Breaking societal beauty standards and embracing natural textures.

- The emotional and mental empowerment of loving your natural hair.

Natural hair is so much more than a trend—it's a statement, a legacy, and a form of resistance. Throughout history, Black women's hair has symbolized our identity, culture, and strength. From the intricate braids of African tribes, each with its own meaning, to the bold Afro movement of the 1960s, natural hair has always been a way for us to express who we are unapologetically.

In the past, Black women were pressured to conform to Eurocentric beauty standards that deemed straight hair "acceptable" and "professional." But as time evolved, so did our perceptions. Today, wearing natural hair is an act of reclaiming our beauty standards. No more hiding curls, coils, or kinks. We embrace our God-given texture with pride, knowing it represents our roots, culture, and history.

Breaking Societal Standards

For far too long, societal standards suggested that beauty was synonymous with straight hair. But natural hair has proven time and time again that beauty comes in all forms. Celebrities like Solange Knowles and Viola Davis have taken a stand with their natural hair, showing the world that our beauty is limitless and diverse. Solange once said, *"I love my hair because it's a reflection of me, and I love me." This message is at the core of what it means to embrace your natural hair—it's about loving yourself exactly as you are.

Emotional and Mental Empowerment

The journey to loving your natural hair isn't just physical; it's deeply emotional and transformative. Transitioning to natural hair means more than just ditching chemical treatments—it's about accepting and loving your authentic self. It's liberating, empowering, and boosts your confidence. When you embrace your natural hair, you're saying to the world, "This is me, and I am enough."

HairLyfe's Mission

At HairLyfe, we understand the emotional and cultural connection Black women have with their hair. That's why we've created a line of products specifically designed to nourish, strengthen, and protect your hair. Our mission is simple: to empower women to embrace their natural beauty with pride. From our restorative Hair Reset Line, every product is formulated with the best natural ingredients to support your hair on this journey of self-love and empowerment.

The Evolution of Natural Hair

Over the decades, natural hair has transformed into a symbol of empowerment. Today, Black women are redefining beauty on their own terms, rocking everything from Afros and twists to Bantu knots and locs with pride. This evolution represents a cultural shift—one where natural hair is not just accepted, but celebrated. As Issa Rae famously said, "My hair is an extension of me. I think it shows that you are comfortable with yourself."

At HairLyfe, we're here to support every step of your journey, ensuring your hair is as healthy and beautiful as you are. Together, we're rewriting the narrative of what it means to wear your hair naturally, boldly, and unapologetically.

Conclusion

Your natural hair is more than just a style—it's a crown, a statement, and a symbol of your strength. By embracing your natural hair, you're embracing your history, your beauty, and your power. At HairLyfe, we are honored to be a part of your journey, offering the products and support you need to nurture your hair and yourself. Join us in celebrating the power of natural hair and let your crown shine.

Embracing Your Unique Crown

Every twist, curl, and coil of natural hair tells a story, one that is uniquely yours. The journey of embracing your natural texture is about rediscovering that individuality. As you move through this journey, remember that your hair isn't just a part of your appearance—it's an extension of your identity, reflecting your heritage and personal growth. In a world that often pushes uniformity, choosing to wear your natural hair is a powerful act of self-expression and pride. It is an affirmation that your natural beauty is enough, and that your hair, in all its glory, deserves to be celebrated.

The Liberation of Authenticity

Transitioning to natural hair can be a liberating experience, both physically and emotionally. For many women, it marks a significant turning point in their lives—a shedding of societal expectations and a reclaiming of their true selves. The process of nurturing your natural hair can be deeply healing, as it requires patience, care, and understanding of your own unique needs. This journey is not just about the hair itself; it's about embracing every part of who you are. When you choose authenticity over conformity, you unlock a deeper connection to yourself, one that radiates confidence and inner strength.

A Journey of Self-Love and Community

At its core, the natural hair movement is about more than just hair care—it's about community, empowerment, and self-love. As more women embrace their natural textures, we create a ripple effect of acceptance and pride within the Black community. It's a reminder that we are not alone on this journey. Our natural hair, in all its diversity, is a shared symbol of our collective strength and resilience. By choosing to honor your natural hair, you are not only reclaiming your own beauty, but you are also uplifting others to do the same. Together, we stand as a testament to the beauty of authenticity and the power of embracing who we truly are.

UNDERSTANDING YOUR HAIR TYPE AND TEXTURE

Welcome to Chapter Two! Now that we've explored the beauty and power of natural hair, it's time to get personal. Understanding your hair's unique characteristics is the first step toward mastering your hair care routine and fully embracing your natural beauty. Let's dive into the fascinating world of hair types, textures, and the individuality that makes your hair truly one-of-a-kind!

Key Topics

- Different Hair Types (3A-4C): Each curl pattern has its own personality, from loose waves to tight coils. Whether you have soft, bouncy curls or kinky, coily strands, your hair type deserves special care.

- Porosity, Density, and Texture: Your hair's ability to absorb moisture (porosity), its thickness (density), and its feel (texture) are just as important as its curl pattern. Knowing these will help you choose the best products and routine for your hair.

- There's No "One-Size-Fits-All" Approach: Your hair is unique, and so is your journey! Let's break free from the idea that there's only one "right" way to care for natural hair.

Breaking Down Hair Types

- **3A-3C:** Loose curls and ringlets, more prone to frizz but easier to define. Needs lightweight products to maintain bounce without weighing curls down.

- **4A-4C:** Tight curls, kinks, and coils, with 4C being the most densely packed. These textures often need heavier, moisture-rich products to combat dryness and promote elasticity.

Myths Debunked

- **Shrinkage:** Your curls may appear shorter after washing due to shrinkage, but this is a sign of healthy, hydrated hair. Don't worry—your hair is thriving!

- **Uniform Curls:** Many believe their hair should curl the same way all over, but most women have more than one curl pattern. Embrace the beauty of your hair's diversity!

How to Embrace Your Unique Hair Texture

Step into the mirror, sis, and admire your hair's unique story! Whether you're rocking loose curls or tightly coiled kinks, every strand is beautiful. It's time to honor your hair with the love and care it deserves. Don't stress about trying to fit into a box—celebrate your individuality, because no two curl patterns are alike.

At HairLyfe, we believe in **honoring your hair's texture** by using products that cater to its specific needs. Our natural ingredients—like shea butter, avocado oil, and castor oil—are designed to hydrate, strengthen, and nourish every curl, coil, and kink.

Embracing your unique texture means understanding that your hair's journey is unlike anyone else's. What works for someone else may not work for you, and that's perfectly okay. Your natural hair is as individual as you are, and finding the right routine is key to unlocking its full potential. Start by listening to your hair—pay attention to how it responds to different products, styles, and techniques. This is a journey of self-discovery and self-love, and with each step, you'll learn more about what makes your crown truly flourish.

Hair care is not just about products; it's about building a relationship with your hair. Take the time to nurture it, be patient with it, and most importantly, be kind to yourself along the way. Whether it's through protective styling, deep conditioning, or simply letting your hair breathe, every decision you make should be rooted in love. At HairLyfe, we're committed to helping you create a hair care routine that honors your texture and empowers you to feel confident and radiant every day.

Consistency is key when it comes to caring for your natural hair. Establishing a regular routine—whether it's weekly wash days, monthly treatments, or daily moisturizing—helps your hair thrive. It's important to remember that healthy hair is happy hair, and the more love you pour into it, the more your curls, kinks, and coils will thank you. Embrace the process and know that the time and care you invest in your hair are acts of self-care and empowerment.

Part of embracing your natural hair texture is learning to be patient with it. Hair growth, texture changes, and achieving your hair goals all take time. It's easy to become discouraged, but remember that your journey is unique, and every stage is worth celebrating. From the early days of transitioning to fully embracing your natural texture, each moment is a step toward becoming more in tune with your authentic self. Trust the process, and enjoy watching your hair evolve and thrive.

Lastly, embrace versatility. Your natural hair gives you the freedom to experiment with styles, textures, and looks that reflect your personality and mood. From sleek and defined curls to bold, voluminous afros, there are endless ways to express yourself through your hair. Don't be afraid to switch it up and have fun with your hair journey. At HairLyfe, we're here to support you with the tools and products to keep your hair healthy and vibrant, no matter how you choose to style it. This journey is all about you—honoring your roots, your beauty, and your crown.

24

BUILDING A NATURAL HAIR CARE ROUTINE

Now that you've embraced your unique hair texture, it's time to craft a routine that nurtures and protects your crown. Building a solid hair care regimen is essential to keeping your natural hair healthy, strong, and radiant. In this chapter, we'll walk you through the key steps, methods, and products that will make caring for your natural hair a joyful and rewarding experience.

Key Topics

- Essential Steps for a Healthy Hair Regimen: Moisturizing, cleansing, and protective styling.

- Frequency Recommendations: How often to wash, deep condition, and detangle based on your hair type.

- Avoiding Common Hair Care Mistakes: Tips for a consistent, effective routine.

Step-by-Step Guide to Creating Your Custom Hair Care Routine

1. Cleansing

A clean scalp is a healthy scalp. Natural hair thrives when it's free of product buildup and excess oils. Depending on your hair type:

- 3A–3C hair types may benefit from washing once a week to maintain volume without drying out curls.

- 4A–4C hair types typically require cleansing every two weeks to avoid stripping the hair of its natural oils.

Use a sulfate-free shampoo, like HairLyfe's Hair Reset Shampoo, which gently cleanses without drying, leaving your hair refreshed and nourished.

2. Deep Conditioning

Hydration is key to healthy curls. Deep condition your hair regularly to restore moisture, repair damage, and promote softness and elasticity. For tighter curls (4A-4C), deep condition every 1-2 weeks, while looser curls (3A-3C) may need it bi-weekly.

Try our Hair Reset Conditioner, an exquisite blend of slippery elm, aloe vera, and BTMS conditioning emulsifiers that deeply nourish, hydrate, and detangle; enriched with black seed oil, moringa, silk, and honey, this luxurious formula envelops each strand, leaving your hair irresistibly soft, radiant, and revitalized.

3. Moisturizing (The LOC Method)

The LOC method—Liquid, Oil, Cream—is the holy grail for locking in moisture. After washing, apply:

- Liquid: Start with water and our HairLyfe Quench Crème Infusion

- Oil: Seal in the moisture our Hair Reset Serum, a twenty plus herbal blend including castor oil, jojoba oil, and peppermint just to name a few.

- Cream: Finish with our Silk Essence Hydrating Custard, or a creamy product to define curls and keep them soft.

This method helps keep hair hydrated for days, reducing breakage and promoting long-term health.

4. Protective Styling

Styles like twists, braids, and buns protect your ends, minimize manipulation, and help retain length. Remember to moisturize and seal your hair before protective styling and protect your edges with HairLyfe Prestige Edge Sculptor.

Recommended Frequency for Wash Days and Care

Washing

- For looser curls (3A–3C): Once a week.

- For tighter curls (4A–4C): Every two weeks or as needed.

Deep Conditioning

- 3A–3C: Every other wash.

- 4A–4C: Every wash or every other wash.

Detangling

- Detangling natural hair requires patience. Use a wide-tooth comb or fingers on damp, conditioned hair to minimize breakage. For kinkier textures, detangle in sections with our HairLyfe Hair Reset Cascade Silk Mist

Common Mistakes to Avoid

- Over-Washing

Washing too often can strip your hair of its natural oils, leaving it dry and brittle. Stick to a schedule that works for your texture and focus on keeping your hair moisturized between washes.

- Skipping Deep Conditioning

Natural hair craves moisture. Skipping deep conditioning sessions can lead to dry, unmanageable hair and increased breakage.

- Using Harsh Products

Avoid products with sulfates, parabens, and synthetic fragrances that can damage your hair and scalp. opt for natural, nourishing ingredients like those found in HairLyfe's all-natural line.

HairLyfe Products Spotlight

- Hair Reset Shampoo: Gently cleanses and hydrates without stripping your hair.

- Hair Reset Conditioning: Restores moisture and strength to curls and coils.

- Hair Reset Serum: A blend of nourishing oils to promote hair growth and lock in moisture.

- HairLyfe Cascade Silk Mist: Softens and smooths hair, making detangling easy.

Your natural hair deserves care that honors its beauty and strength. By building a routine that focuses on moisture, protection, and consistent love, you'll see your hair thrive! Ready to start your journey? Shop our products at myhairlyfe.com and follow us @shophairlyfe for tips, inspiration, and product guides.

CHAPTER FOUR

CHOOSING THE RIGHT NATURAL HAIR PRODUCTS

Choosing the right products for your natural hair can be overwhelming, but with the right knowledge, you'll feel empowered to make informed decisions that support your hair's health and beauty. In this chapter, we'll guide you through understanding product labels, avoiding harmful ingredients, and selecting natural products that nurture your hair's unique needs.

Key Topics

- **Reading Labels & Avoiding Harmful Ingredients:** What to avoid and why.

- **Benefits of Natural & Organic Ingredients:** How nature can elevate your hair care routine.

- **Choosing the Right Products:** What to look for in shampoos, conditioners, oils, and treatments based on your hair goals.

How to Read Product Labels and Avoid Harmful Ingredients

When choosing hair products, the ingredients list can tell you everything you need to know. Keep an eye out for harmful chemicals that can damage your hair over time.

Avoid These Ingredients

- **Sulfates**: Harsh detergents found in many shampoos that strip the hair of natural oils, leaving it dry and prone to breakage.

- **Parabens**: Preservatives that can disrupt hormonal balance and irritate the scalp.

- **Silicones**: These create a synthetic shine but often lead to product buildup, blocking moisture from penetrating the hair shaft.

- **Synthetic Fragrances & Dyes**: These can irritate the scalp and damage hair with repeated use.

Choose Products with Natural Ingredients

- **Aloe Vera**: Soothes the scalp and locks in moisture.

- **Shea Butter**: A rich moisturizer that provides deep hydration and protects against breakage.

- **Coconut Oil**: Penetrates the hair shaft to strengthen and nourish from within.

- **Castor Oil**: Known for promoting hair growth and improving hair thickness.

- **Avocado Oil**: Lightweight yet deeply nourishing, perfect for softening and adding shine.

Why Natural Products Are Better for Your Hair Health

Your hair is as unique as you are, and it deserves products that work with its natural chemistry—not against it. Products packed with natural, organic ingredients are more compatible with your hair's needs, promoting long-term health, growth, and shine.

- **Growth**: Ingredients like castor oil and rosemary oil stimulate hair follicles and improve blood circulation to the scalp, encouraging healthy growth.

- **Volume**: Lightweight oils like avocado and grapeseed oil add volume without weighing down your hair, leaving your curls full of life.

- **Hydration**: Natural butters and oils (shea butter, olive oil) deeply moisturize the hair, making it more manageable and less prone to frizz and breakage.

HairLyfe Products Spotlight

At HairLyfe, we've crafted a line of natural hair care products designed to nourish, protect, and elevate your curls, coils, and kinks. Our ingredients are carefully selected to ensure your hair gets only the best nature has to offer.

- **HairLyfe Hair Reset Shampoo**: Featuring nourishing ingredients like shea butter, honeyquat, and botanical extracts, including hibiscus and ginseng, to cleanse, hydrate, and rejuvenate for luxurious, healthy lock.

- **HairLyfe Hair Reset Conditioner**: An exquisite blend of slippery elm, aloe vera, and BTMS conditioning emulsifiers that deeply nourish, hydrate, and detangle; enriched with black seed oil, moringa, silk, and honey, this luxurious formula envelops each strand, leaving your hair irresistibly soft, radiant, and revitalized.

- **HairLyfe Hair Reset Serum**: a luxurious blend of sunflower, chebe, fenugreek, and almond oil, peppermint, rosemary, nourishing each strand for unparalleled shine and vitality while promoting healthy growth and strength.

- **HairLyfe Hair Reset Cascade Silk Mist**: A luxurious blend of organic aloe leaf juice, coconut oil, shea butter, and cocoa butter, enriched with pro-vitamin B5 and Madagascar vanilla extract, designed to deeply hydrate, nourish, and revitalize your hair for unmatched softness and shine.

Tips for Selecting Products Based on Hair Goals

- **For Growth**: Look for products containing ingredients like castor oil, peppermint, and rosemary oil that stimulate the scalp and support hair growth.

- **For Volume**: Lightweight oils and volumizing creams that won't weigh down your curls are key. Look for avocado oil and grapeseed oil.

- **For Hydration**: Deep conditioners and leave-in treatments with shea butter, coconut oil, and honey will provide the moisture your hair craves.

Your natural hair deserves products that are as luxurious and unique as you are. By understanding what to look for in product labels and selecting ingredients that nurture your hair's health, you're setting yourself up for a lifetime of healthy, thriving hair. Ready to upgrade your routine? Explore HairLyfe's all-natural collection and give your hair the love it deserves at **myhairlyfe.com**.

When it comes to your hair, quality matters. Each strand is a testament to your unique beauty, and the products you choose should reflect that. At HairLyfe, we understand that natural hair needs more than just hydration—it requires thoughtful, intentional care. Our formulas are meticulously crafted with high-quality, all-natural ingredients that not only nourish but also enhance the strength and vitality of your hair.

From moisturizing leave-ins to hydrating serums, each product in our collection is designed to target the specific needs of natural hair. Whether you're battling dryness, looking to define your curls, or seeking to boost growth, HairLyfe's range has a solution tailored just for you. With every use, your hair will feel more manageable, softer, and more vibrant—because when your hair thrives, so do you.

It's not just about the products, though. The journey to healthy, flourishing hair starts with self-awareness and embracing your natural beauty in all its forms. Your hair is your crown, and every step you take in your natural hair care routine is a form of self-love and empowerment. That's why at HairLyfe, we're committed to supporting you with more than just products; we offer guidance, tips, and education to help you make informed choices for your hair's long-term health.

As you continue on your natural hair journey, remember that every strand, curl, and coil tell a story—one of resilience, beauty, and empowerment. With HairLyfe by your side, you'll have the tools, knowledge, and support to ensure your crown shines as brilliantly as you do. Visit myhairlyfe.com today, and start treating your hair with the luxury it deserves. Your journey to vibrant, healthy hair begins now!

CHAPTER FIVE

PROTECTIVE STYLES, GROWTH, AND LONG-TERM HAIR HEALTH

Protective styles are an essential tool in any natural hair journey, offering a way to maintain hair health while encouraging growth. In this chapter, we will explore how to incorporate protective styles into your routine, tips for transitioning from relaxed to natural hair, and how to preserve the integrity of your hair for long-term growth and health.

Key Topics

- Importance of Protective Styles: How braids, twists, and buns protect hair.

- Transitioning from Relaxed to Natural Hair: A gentle approach to going natural.

- Retaining Length and Avoiding Breakage: Best practices to keep hair strong.

The Importance of Protective Styles

Protective styles like braids, twists, buns, and updos are not only fashionable but also key to promoting hair growth and preserving the health of your strands. By tucking your ends away, protective styles minimize exposure to the elements, reducing breakage and split ends caused by daily wear and tear.

Popular Protective Styles

Box braids, cornrows, faux locs, and Bantu knots are among the most popular protective styles for natural hair. These styles can be worn for extended periods, allowing your hair to rest and thrive.

Benefits of Protective Styles

Not only do they shield your hair from environmental damage, but protective styles also give your hair the chance to grow longer and stronger by reducing manipulation.

Tips for Transitioning from Relaxed to Natural Hair

Transitioning to natural hair is a deeply personal experience, and protective styles can make the process easier by reducing the need for frequent manipulation of two different textures.

Protective Styles for Transitioning

Styles like flat twists, box braids, or wigs can help manage the transition while minimizing heat and chemical damage. These styles allow the natural hair to grow out while protecting the relaxed ends.

Trim Regularly

Gradually trim the relaxed ends over time to ensure your natural curls remain healthy. Don't rush the process—your hair will thank you!

Retaining Length and Avoiding Breakage

One of the biggest challenges in growing natural hair is retaining length. Protective styling is only effective if accompanied by good hair care practices.

- Moisturize Regularly: Even while in a protective style, your hair needs moisture. Use our hydrating *Hair Reset Cascade Silk Mist*.

- Protect Your Edges: Edges are often the most delicate part of natural hair. Avoid tight braids or styles that pull on your edges. To maintain growth, apply our Prestige Edge Sculptor to nourish and protect them.

Conclusion: Your Hair, Your Crown

Your natural hair is more than just a style—it's a reflection of your identity, strength, and beauty. Whether you're rocking protective styles, defining your curls, or transitioning from relaxed hair, remember that your hair is your crown, deserving of love and care every step of the way.

Join the HairLyfe community on social media @shophairlyfe for daily inspiration, hair care tips, and exclusive offers that empower you to embrace your natural hair journey. As a special thank you for reading, enjoy 20% off your next HairLyfe purchase with the code CROWN20.

Your journey to healthy, natural hair is just beginning—let HairLyfe be your guide. Embrace your crown, and wear it proudly. Shop now at myhairlyfe.com.

For more hair care tips, tutorials, and inspiration, be sure to explore our full range of resources below. HairLyfe is here to support you every step of the way on your natural hair journey!

Our website: www.myhairlyfe.com

Explore our full range of natural hair products, read our latest blog posts, and shop exclusive deals on myhairlyfe.com

Follow HairLyfe on social media! Instagram, Facebook TikTok: @shophairlyfe

Exclusive Offer

Don't forget to use your promo code "CROWN20" for 20% off your next purchase on myhairlyfe.com!